COCONUT OIL
THE "NEW" SUPERFOOD

THE *5 KEY* COCONUT OIL BENEFITS
YOU NEED TO KNOW ABOUT

 FOR VIBRANT HEALTH, RADIANT BEAUTY AND WEIGHT LOSS

Disclaimer

Introduction

You're exhausted. This feeling, this aching tiredness you're feeling: you understand that everyone you know struggles with it. They struggle with signs of aging, with wrinkles sagging beneath their eyes, just like you. You buy all the proper anti-aging, chemically advanced creams—these creams even recommended by dermatologists and doctors. And you search for the proper weight supplements in order to reduce your waist size. You diet and exercise with futility; it seems there's nothing you can do to escape this aging game. You will simply never feel like yourself again; you're sure.

But this has been happening to generation after generation, to population upon population, for as long as humans have lived on earth, you think. Why should yours be any different? It's best to accept the worst.

Looking back, however, this acceptance of bitter aging and weight gain is not how many humans lived. They lived vibrantly in tropical locations with youthful faces, thin waistlines, and bright, lively hair. They lived out loud, in the sun on the beach. In the shadows of their livelihood: the palm tree. And from the palm tree hung their true grail: the coconut.

The insides of the coconut yield coconut milk and meat. However, when the coconut meat is pressed just right, it relinquishes oil. And this coconut oil is the master behind the wonderful livelihood of these thousand year old populations. These civilizations used it for everything. They cooked with it. They washed with it—their hair, their face, everything. They utilized it to treat digestive, bacterial, and other health problems. And they lived well with this natural product they plucked directly from the trees above them. They had no real body problems. They had all they needed.

Coconut oil has come back in style in the past several years, but it is not like the fleeting "reduce aging" or "lose weight" scams of past styles. It is not a here today, gone tomorrow situation. Coconut oil comes in its natural state; it contains no hormone-altering chemicals. It revs your metabolism, reduces aging, and makes you a more full, complete, healthy person.

Understand the true health benefits behind coconut oil: how it works, why it works, and the ways in which your life will change. Do not hesitate to administer the natural remedy of coconut oil into your everyday routine. It is from the earth; it is waiting for you.

Table of Contents

Introduction 3

CHAPTER 1
FACTS AND FICTIONS OF COCONUT OIL: THE
TRUTH BEHIND THE TROPICAL SERUM 7

Coconut Oil Formation Process 7

Coconut Oil at a Molecular Level................................. 8

Coconut Oil Benefits 11

CHAPTER 2
A HEALING AGENT: THE REAL HEALTH BENEFITS
OF COCONUT OIL 12

Boost Your Immunity 13

Resist Candida Yeast Infections 14

Create a Hormonal Balance 15

CHAPTER 3
BYE BYE SUGAR CRAVINGS: WEIGHT LOSS AND
COCONUT OIL 16

Boost Your Metabolism 16

Fight Back Against Type 2 Diabetes 16

Control Your Weight, Assist Your Weight Loss Goals,
and Eliminate Further Sugar Cravings 18

Irresistible Coconut Oil Raspberry and Strawberry
Smoothie 19

CHAPTER 4
BEAUTIFUL HAIR: COCONUT OIL FOR RADIANT
HAIR AND SCALP **20**

Create a Healthy Scalp Routine 20

Alleviate an Itchy Scalp 21

Tea Tree Coconut Oil Scalp Treatment Recipe 21

Citrus Coconut Oil Scalp Treatment Recipe 23

Boost Hair Shine and Strength with Coconut Oil
Deep Conditioning 23

Coconut Oil and Raw Honey Deep Conditioning
Mask Recipe 24

CHAPTER 5
YOU LOOK SO YOUNG: FIGHT WRINKLES, AGE
SPOTS, BUG BITES WITH COCONUT OIL SKIN
REMEDIES **25**

Fight the Aging Process: Reduce Wrinkles and Age
Spots 25

Anti-Aging Coconut Oil Facial Skin Cream 26

Makeup Removers 27

Bug Bite Busters 27

Coconut Oil Based Bug Repellant 28

Conclusion 30

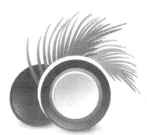

CHAPTER 1

FATS AND FICTIONS OF COCONUT OIL:
The Truth Behind the Tropical Serum

That fuzzy fruit ball hanging from the tall, tropical tree at the beach doesn't look so life affirming at first glance. Bust it open, however, and you have a medicinal remedy, a weight loss supplement, a digestive, a metabolizer, and excellent cooking oil. Coconut oil has been utilized over the entire world for thousands of years; a 1950's document published in the United States, however, refuted the thousand-year-old renowned effects, proclaiming the coconut oil to be cholesterol boosting. The scare-tactics utilized by this 1950's study were falsely wrought, taking humans away from the natural force found in the heart of the coconut. The health effects speak for themselves through a closer look at the molecular formation and benefits of creating a coconut oil-filled lifestyle.

Coconut Oil Formation Process
Coconut oil is extracted from the meat in the coconut; the hard, hairy shell is stripped from the meat, leaving the white meat behind. The processes varied over the years of coconut usage.

However, oftentimes the meat is shredded and then allowed to dry out to ten percent moisture. After the drying process is complete, one utilizes a manual press to literally squeeze the oil from the meat. Other processes involve screw presses. Approximately seventy liters of coconut oil can be extracted from 1,440 kilograms of full coconuts.

Coconut Oil at a Molecular Level

Coconut oil is filled with saturated fatty acids. This sounds terrifying to health nuts everywhere; but before writing coconut oil off as unhealthy, it's best to understand the saturated fats contained in coconut oil at the molecular level.

There are several versions of the saturated fats you digest every day; and it's true that a high level of saturated fat in the blood stream is a hindrance to your health—resulting in high cholesterol and heart disease. However, the truth of coconut oil saturated fat results in quite the opposite bodily reaction.

Essentially, the difference between coconut oil saturated fats and the saturated fats in consumed animal fat and oil seed fats lies in the carbon atom count at the molecular level. Animal fat saturated fatty acids contain up to eighteen carbon atoms while the coconut oil fatty acid has, at the most, twelve, and at the least, eight. Therefore, the fatty acids in the coconut oil are referred to as short and medium fatty acids, or short and medium chain triglycerides (rather than large fatty acids or triglycerides). These shorter chains of triglycerides contribute to a variety of health benefits, altering various mechanics in your body at this cellular level: they help to reduce cholesterol, fight Alzheimer's disease, and assist with gall bladder and liver diseases.

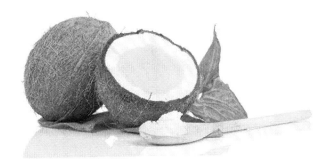

Immediately upon your body's consumption and digestion of coconut oil, the coconut oil proceeds to your liver. This is because your body cannot utilize anything but straight glucose as a form of energy—and glucose is only found in carbohydrates. Therefore, your liver must convert the fatty acids in the digested coconut oil into glucose during the complicated Kreb's Cycle. Essentially, your body utilizes many more calories, revving your metabolism, in order to utilize the energy contained in the coconut oil. Best of all: the calories found in the digested coconut oil are not directed into fat cells, ready to bring your weight down.

The short fatty acid chains in coconut oil are unlike that enemy, the trans fatty acids, in that once trans fatty acids are digested and converted, your body isn't sure how to utilize them for energy. This is because the "trans fatty acid chains" have been chemically altered; the hydrogen in the connecting chains has been placed differently, thus allowing whatever food they make up to have a greater shelf life. This forces your body to treat the fatty acid chains differently. Therefore, while the saturated fatty acids in your coconut oil goes to assist your brain function, your heart health, and your digestion, trans fatty acids go—essentially nowhere. But they're stuck in your body after digestion. They end up building up on your blood vessels and your brain lining, affecting proper communication between cells.

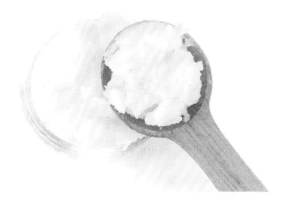

Coconut Oil Benefits

Cooking with these short and medium fatty acid chains found in coconut oil allows for several benefits outlined in the following chapters. It boosts your metabolism via the transfer from lipids to body-utilizing glucose. It alleviates Type 2 Diabetes, and it acts as an antibiotic against your body's intruders. Therefore, any saturated fat fear you retain must be purged; the ancient tropical peoples across the world survived their various climates, their ancient diseases by utilizing this natural product. Do not refute this remedy.

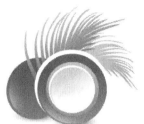

CHAPTER 2

A HEALING AGENT:
The Real Health Benefits of Coconut Oil

Inflammation in your digestive health, be it just a brief disruption or a more serious disease, like Crohn's disease, is an all out rage against your daily life. If your body cannot digest the food you intake each day, you cannot naturally receive the caloric benefits of your food; you cannot grow new muscle, grow new brain cell tissue, or have enough energy for proper cell-to-cell communication. Not only that: your stomach is bloated, you feel unattractive and 'under the weather' nearly all the time. Usually, bacteria, candida, or parasites are involved in the disruption, oftentimes causing ulcers.

Luckily, the short and medium sized fatty acids found in coconut oil assist with your digestive disorders. They are digested quite differently than most carbohydrates and long chain fatty acids. The chains are obviously smaller and therefore require less enzymes and less digestive energy in order to break them down. Because these medium chain fatty acids are broken down so quickly, your pancreatic juices do not have to enter into the equation, thus putting no strain on your pancreas. Usually, your pancreas is incredibly overworked when you eat fat. Furthermore, after initial digestion in your digestive tract, the medium chain fatty acids do not need to be packaged in order to be distributed throughout your body like large chain fatty acids. Your medium chain fatty acids are deposited directly to your liver for transfer from fat to glucose. Therefore, the nutrients are easily assimilated into energy for your body without expending the digestive energy to package them.

Eating coconut oil in order to give your digestive system a break is especially beneficial as you age. Your digestive system, unfortunately, ages along with the rest of you; it is unable to make as many fat-burning enzymes. Therefore, maintaining coconut oil in your system requires less of these enzymes while administering the proper fat intake for continued energy.

Boost Your Immunity

Coconut oil is fueled with many body-beneficial fats such as lauric acid, capylic acid, and capric acids: all of these acids contain elements that work against bacteria, fungus, and virus growth in your body cells. Lauric acid, in particular, makes up approximately fifty percent of coconut oil. In the conversion process in the liver after initial digestion, coconut oils' lauric acid is switched to monolaurin. Monolaurin is actually a property found in mother's breast milk; it acts as an anti-bacterial element, protecting the baby from harm in the early stages, when he or she cannot protect him or herself from the raging surrounding bacteria without a strong immunity. Therefore, utilizing coconut oil is much like boosting your immunity when you were a baby; monolaurin actually destroys the cell membranes of microbes, eliminating them from your system.

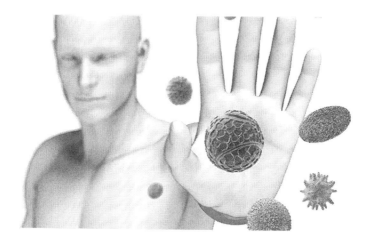

Resist Candida Yeast Infections

Yeast naturally occurs in your digestive system; healthy people produce enough good bacteria to gobble up the extra yeast, thus forcing a yeast balance. Unfortunately, yeast production can get out of control incredibly easily: especially if you have a poor diet, if you're on specific kinds of birth control, or if you're stressed. If you suffer from yeast infections, coconut oil is easily one of the best medicinal remedies. Look once again to the lauric and capylic acids; after their transfer in the liver, lauric acid and capylic acid have been found to penetrate yeast membranes throughout the digestive system, thus killing them. Thus, coconut oil has been found to be one of the most beneficial digestive detox remedies in the world.

Create a Hormonal Balance

Several every day products you utilize for your face, hair, and nutrition contain harmful chemicals; these chemicals actually alter your hormonal balance. Switching to coconut based facial cleansers and make up removers can easily eliminate these hormonal imbalances. A hormonal imbalanced nutritional example lies in soy and soy-based oils, often thought to be beneficial for nutrition. Unfortunately, soy-based products alter your thyroid functions, therefore slowing your metabolism to a slow crawl. An increase in coconut oil medium chain fatty acids boosts your metabolism and revs your thyroid to act correctly. Furthermore, these medium chain fatty acids actually increase your interior body temperature. An increased body temperature allows for a proper metabolism; it assists in pushing your thyroid to proper functionality.

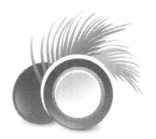

CHAPTER 3

BYE BYE SUGAR CRAVINGS:
Weight Loss and Coconut Oil

Boost Your Metabolism

At the beginning of a diet plan, its best to begin by supplementing your diet with the best natural weight loss supplement: coconut oil. Whenever you eat anything, approximately ten percent of the calories you consume must be utilized in order to digest and convert the food to appropriate energy. As aforementioned, coconut oil is rich in medium chain fatty acids that actually force your body to utilize a bit more energy, thus revving your ten percent caloric usage of the foods you eat to about fifteen percent. In turn, this boosts your metabolism, turns your body temperature up a few notches, and pushes your thyroid glands to work properly. A properly functioning thyroid gland easily promotes weight loss and enhanced metabolism.

Fight Back Against Type 2 Diabetes

High fat, high sugar diets yield high Type 2 Diabetes rates. For example, approximately ten percent of the United States' population is affected with Type 2 Diabetes. When you eat sugar, your insulin levels go up, forcing the glucose level in your blood to reduce. Glucose is, of course, necessary for proper energy and brain function, and insulin is necessary in order to tackle the glucose, forcing it to appropriate areas throughout the body. When someone has Type 2 Diabetes, however, his or her blood is insulin resistant. Therefore, the body produces too much insulin to send into the blood stream to deal with glucose levels. A high level of insulin in the blood is incredibly dangerous.

In order to counteract the effects of this insulin resistance, diabetics stay far away from sugar. However, if you eat your carbohydrates with a bit of coconut oil, your body and blood stream are not attacked with the sugar all at once. Instead, coconut oil forces the body to slow the digestive process; energy passes coolly through your system without giving you a spike and then a dangerous drop. Furthermore, long-chain fatty acids found in other cooking oils, like sunflower oil, actually promotes fat storage. This fat storage decreases your body's ability to absorb sugar from the blood stream, thus leaving extra glucose out to dry. Therefore, your body has to handle this excess blood sugar by transmitting still more insulin into your stream. This can contribute to a strong insulin resistance.

Furthermore, the increased metabolic rate created with the addition of coconut oil in your diet creates a healthier, more revving you: one more susceptible to weight loss. Without the additional sugar and fat cells, your body will have the ability to withstand greater amounts of glucose with a higher insulin sensitivity.

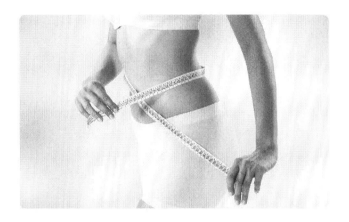

Control Your Weight, Assist Your Weight Loss Goals, and Eliminate Further Sugar Cravings

Essentially, weight loss is the result of fewer calories in, more calories expended. Sounds simple, but as any struggling human on the planet knows, it's just not. However, incorporating coconut oil into your diet can eliminate sugar cravings and help you reach your weight loss goals. Coconut oil revs your metabolism through its boost of your body's temperature and through its unusual conversion: straight from your digestive tract to your liver. Unlike most long chain fatty acids, it does not sit well pre-packaged, ready for storage in your body (and, unattractively, on your belly). Furthermore, upon digestion and conversion in your liver, coconut oil is transferred to ketone bodies. Ketone bodies are an excellent appetite reducer, thus allowing you to eat much less throughout the day.

Of course, it's best to understand that a diet and exercise regime along with the coconut oil administration will create the best weight loss strategy. A diet low in carbohydrates, high in protein, and full with the coconut oil benefits will allow you to reduce dangerous abdominal fat, increase your insulin sensitivity, and rev your metabolism.

Try This Delicious, Coconut Oil Rich Dessert for your Next Healthy Sweet Treat:

Irresistible Coconut Oil Raspberry and Strawberry Smoothie

Makes 1 Smoothie.

Ingredients:

1 tbsp. raw virgin coconut oil

½ cup strawberries

½ cup raspberries

1 cup unsweetened vanilla flavored almond milk

5 ice cubes

Directions:

Add your raw virgin coconut oil, your strawberries, your raspberries, your almond milk, and your ice cubes to a blender. Blend on high for a minute and a half or until desired smoothness. Now: beat back against those sugar cravings and enjoy your fibrous, healthy snack!

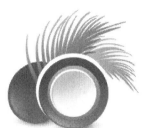

CHAPTER 4

Coconut oil is perfect for you hair care regime at a very molecular level. While most hair care ointments, creams, and shampoos contain fats and oils, they are filled with the aforementioned long chain fatty acids. These long chain fatty acids are too large to assimilate into your hairs; therefore, they simply sit on top of your hair, forcing a sort of cake-y build up over time. This can actually block your follicles and create a lack of hair growth. The medium chain fatty acids of the coconut oil can actually assimilate with your hairs and hair follicles, repairing from the inside out. The lauric acid restructures the hair follicle, trapping the much-needed protein in the strands, allowing for prolonged hair health.

Create a Healthy Scalp Routine

You clip your toenails, maintain your teeth, clean behind your ears; you make sure that every inch of your body is squeaky. And yet, you probably forget your scalp: that thing hiding beneath your hair. It's easy to forget, of course. However, avoiding proper scalp treatment can cause some serious issues: sebum, a hard product build up from all those gels and shampoos can actually clog your hair follicles, thus causing scaling and hair thinning. Furthermore, proper scalp treatments prevent dandruff, stimulate your scalp to promote hair growth from your follicles, and remove all that unnecessary dry flakes from long, dry winters.

Alleviate an Itchy Scalp

An itchy scalp lends no relief. There are many oil or cream-based ointments at various pharmacies; but these tend to contain a variety of hormone-unbalancing chemicals. In fact, research estimates that women imbibe approximately five pounds of chemicals through lotions, creams, and make ups through one year of beauty regime. It's best, when relying on skin creams, to rely on natural remedies in order to not create havoc on your insides. Remember: your skin—including your scalp—is the greatest organ of your body. Anything you put on it is transmitted to your interior.

Tea Tree Coconut Oil Scalp Treatment Recipe

Ingredients:
4 tbsp. coconut oil
4 drops tea tree oil
4 drops rosemary oil
Nylon application brush

Directions:

Begin by mixing your coconut oil, tea tree oil, and rosemary oil together in a small bowl. Utilize the dry nylon application brush and rotate the brush along the scalp while pressing firmly down. Repeat, making sure to part your hair and diving appropriately close to your skin. Pressing firmly—but not too hard—stimulates the blood circulation to your scalp. Next, utilize the same nylon brush and apply the mixture. Work in one-inch sections throughout your head. Leave the treatment in your hair for twenty minutes; ask someone to rub your scalp during this time for added relaxation. Rinse.

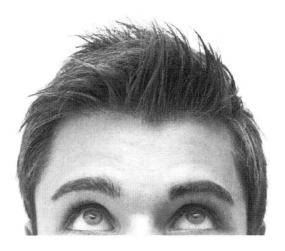

Citrus Coconut Oil Scalp Treatment Recipe

Ingredients:

4 tbsp. coconut oil

2 tbsp. lemon juice

1 tbsp. grapefruit juice

Directions:

Begin by mixing your coconut oil, lemon juice, and grapefruit juice together in a small bowl. Utilize the dry nylon application brush and rotate the brush along the scalp while pressing firmly down. Repeat, making sure to part your hair and diving appropriately close to your skin. Pressing firmly—but not too hard—stimulates the blood circulation to your scalp. Next, utilize the same nylon brush and apply the mixture. Work in one-inch sections throughout your head. Leave the treatment in your hair for twenty minutes; ask someone to rub your scalp during this time for added relaxation. Rinse.

Boost Hair Shine and Strength with Coconut Oil Deep Conditioning

All that blow dryer damage and shampoo, gel build up can leave your hair easily tangled and mangled. Coconut oil provides a wonderful base for which to create a remarkable hair mask, one that will alleviate all past damages and prevent future damages from weather and blow dryers. As aforementioned, coconut oil is filled with medium fatty acid chains that easily assimilate into your hair strands; it repairs your hair from the inside, retaining moisture and inducing great shine.

Coconut Oil and Raw Honey Deep Conditioning Mask Recipe

Ingredients:

2 tbsp. coconut oil
1 tbsp. raw honey
Sauce pan

Directions:

Mix your coconut oil and your raw honey together in a saucepan. Heat the mixture for ten minutes on low, stirring continuously. It's important to heat the mask in order to allow your hair follicles to open, thus relieving any gel or shampoo build up.

Section your damp hair into easily manageable increments. Apply the mixture to your damp hair, starting at the top. Be sure to apply it generously to your ends, where most of the blow drying and hair styling damage has occurred. Next, wrap your hair into a high bun and wait for forty-five minutes for the mask to exfoliate. Rinse your hair out in the shower and prepare yourself for easy, beautiful, natural shine.

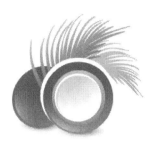

CHAPTER 5
YOU LOOK SO YOUNG:
Fight Wrinkles, Age Spots, Bug Bites with Coconut Oil Skin Remedies

Fight the Aging Process: Reduce Wrinkles and Age Spots

The root of the aging and wrinkle process lies at the cellular level—and can be alleviated, of course, via the medium fatty acid chains of coconut oil. The aging process begins when your exterior facial cells begin to lose their moisture. Essentially, your cell membranes begin to harden, thus removing your cell's ability to receive appropriate amounts of water and nutrients. When your cell parts—like your DNA producing nucleus, for example—don't receive all the necessary water and nutrients, they begin to wither. Furthermore, the processes that occur in your cell—like the aforementioned DNA production—actually produces a great deal of waste called "free radicals." When your cell membrane hardens, your cell is no longer able to expel many of these free radicals. Thus, your cell poisons itself from the inside out. The appearance of wrinkles is due to this strange, self-mutilation at the cellular level.

25

However, when your skin absorbs coconut oil, the medium chain fatty acids are able to position themselves along the cell membrane, repairing and loosening it. Therefore, any cells in the process of poisoning themselves can rectify the situation. Cells can begin receiving moisture once again. It's important to note that other oils and creams with the large chain fatty acids cannot alleviate this problem quite as well; the medium chain fatty acids are the proper size to assimilate perfectly with your cell's membranes.

Anti-Aging Coconut Oil Facial Skin Cream

Ingredients:
¼ cup almond oil
2 tbsp. coconut oil
2 tbsp. beeswax
½ tsp. vitamin E oil
1 tbsp. shea butter

Directions:
Bring a pot of 2 cups of water to a boil. Place all the ingredients: your almond oil, your coconut oil, your beeswax, your vitamin E oil, and your shea oil in a glass jar. When the water has begun to boil, place the glass jar into the boiling water. Stir the mixture occasionally, waiting for it to melt. After it's melted, be sure that everything has combined evenly. Remove it from the boiling water. Allow the jar to sit, uncovered, until the cream cools and solidifies. Close the lid and store in a cool, unlit place.

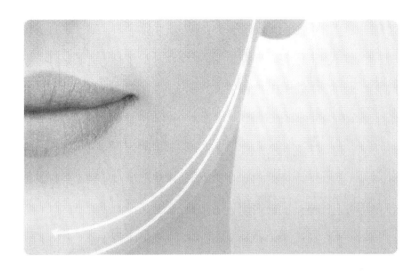

Makeup Removers

Traditional makeup removers, much like anti-aging creams, are ripe with chemicals. Fortunately, in order to remove eye makeup and foundation, you can simply invest in a bit of coconut oil. Put a bit of coconut oil on a cotton ball and smear it over your makeup. Best of all: the minute you administer coconut oil to your face, the medium fatty acids slip into your facial cells, thus adding increased cell health. Therefore, not only are you removing your makeup, you're also assisting in an anti-aging process.

Bug Bite Busters

Bug repellant is fueled with various hormone-disrupting chemicals dangerous for many parts of your body, including your thyroid. If your hormones become imbalanced, you could suffer a whole list of ailments including weight gain, acne, and depression. Essentially, your choice between itchy, scratchy bug bites and bug-spray caused depression is an easy one.

However, you don't have to choose with an incredibly easy coconut oil based bug repellant recipe. The bug bite repellant is not a strange, chemical-smelling spray. It's more like a creamy salve, comfortable to administer to your skin.

Coconut Oil Based Bug Repellant
Makes ½ cup bug balm.

Ingredients:
¼ cup coconut oil
1/8 cup Shea butter
4 tsp. beeswax granules
12 drops citronella essential oil
8 drops rosemary essential oil
8 drops cedar wood essential oil
8 drops lemongrass essential oil
8 drops tea tree essential oil

Tools:
Double boiler
Metal whisk
Metal spoon
jars to deposit completed salve

Directions:
Add water to your double boiler and bring it to a boil. Once it begins boiling, lower the heat to

medium-low. Add the coconut oil and the Shea butter to the top of the double boiler, allowing them to melt together. Continue to whisk throughout. Next, add the beeswax and whisk. Wait until the mixture is completely melted together.

It's now time to test the mixture's texture in order to assure you've proceeded correctly. Dip the back of the metal spoon into the melted liquid. Remove the spoon, allowing the melted mixture to cool and almost solidify into its more creamy texture. Rub it on your hand. If you'd like the texture to be firmer, you can add a bit more beeswax. (Be sure to add it only a ½ tsp. a time.) If you'd like it a bit softer, add some more Shea butter. Once you've reached your desired texture, remove the salve from the heat. After it's cooled for about five minutes, whisk in your essential oils until combined. You can deposit your salve into the prepared jars, but be sure not to cap them until it's completely cooled. Store at room temperature.

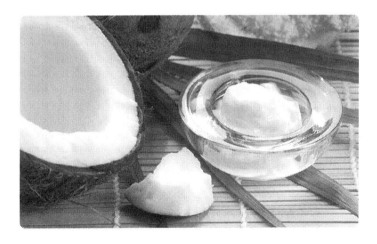

Conclusion

Coconut Oil: The Life-Affirming Tropical Serum Ready to Boost Your Health, Reduce Signs of Aging, and Decrease Your Waist Size has allowed you to understand the truth about coconut oil, at its core. It is fueled with saturated fats; saturated fats that you have been taught to religiously avoid. However, these coconut oil saturated fats contain medium chain fatty acids, fatty acids easily digestible in your system. They enter your liver immediately, ready to transfer into easy energy without forming into easily stored packets of fat: the packets of fat connected to belly fat, thigh fat, that which you're trying to rid yourself. And they don't expel too much digestive energy, therefore allowing your digestive tract to rest while receiving proper energy to repair. Furthermore, when transferred from fat to easily-utilized glucose in your liver, coconut oil fatty acids actually utilize even more calories than most food, thus revving your metabolism and allowing you to lose extra weight.

On a more exterior level, coconut oil does wonders to your hair strands and follicles, removing any gel and shampoo build up. The medium chain fatty acids actually enter the strands, repairing the insides and maintaining the interior proteins. The interior protein allows added shine, thus reducing your need for expensive, chemically altered shiny hair serums.

Coconut oil reduces signs of aging, as well, with its moisture rejuvenation on a cellular level. It repairs your facial cell membranes, allowing them to rid themselves of poisonous free radicals and to accept moisture. Furthermore, coconut oil is a fine, natural ingredient to take the place of bug repellant; no need to utilize smelly, chemically advanced bug spray on your evenings outside.

Coconut oil is the only real remedy you need in order to maintain and reduce your waist size, decrease your sugar cravings, boost real shine to your hair, and give yourself a real, wrinkle-free makeover. Understand the ways in which ancient civilizations lived and thrived; say no to the scientific, chemical advancements on store shelves everywhere. Your answer to prolonged health and happiness lies at the heart of a coconut!

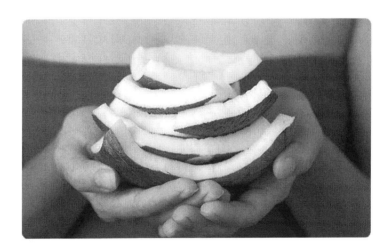

Printed in Great Britain
by Amazon.co.uk, Ltd.,
Marston Gate.